I0390413

Alzheimer's Home Care Guide
"Keys Of Cope"

Written By Elaine Kleid

Published On Createspace

INTRODUCTION

Communicating with people that have Alzheimer's is very different than having a normal everyday conversation. I would describe a conversation with an Alzheimer's patient as random because people with Alzheimer's often say and do very random things.

In order to deal with them effectively, it is important that you try to understand things from their perspective, instead of reacting to what they are saying or doing. This may seem strange, but it is better if you reason with them. Even though their reasoning is often very flawed.

I have written this book to provide you with information I gained during my experience as a caregiver of Alzheimer's patients. I have written this so you can have the tools needed to assist someone that has Alzheimer's, whether it's a family member, friend or even a stranger, without having to read a book of 500 pages or more because that is what I was given to read. So I decided I would like to save you the emotional turmoil of struggling to find out what to do. There are some key things I learned as a caregiver that will help you to deal and interact with those who are affected by Alzheimer's.

TOPICS COVERED

- ➢ Erasing Memories And Its' Changes
- ➢ Communication
- ➢ Identifying Behavioral Triggers
- ➢ Fixation
- ➢ Validating Emotions
- ➢ Identifying Triggers
- ➢ Hygiene
- ➢ Pets
- ➢ Medication Issues
- ➢ Protection Measures (Support System)
- ➢ Embracing The Funny Moments
- ➢ Tips For Caregiver Professionals
- ➢ Time Management
- ➢ Presentation & Organization
- ➢ Enhance Productivity
- ➢ Positive Focus
- ➢ Reaching Out For Help
- ➢ Avoiding Violent Triggers (Preventing Violent Behavior)
- ➢ Arranging Care

When The One You Love Forgets You

Alzheimer's diagnosis typically means that memories will slowly be erased. For some, this devastating disease becomes the main focus of their grief. My hope is to help you focus on the moments you share rather than on what your loved one cannot do or remember anymore.

Be Prepared For Changes In Your Life

Once Alzheimer's is diagnosed, you will notice the person begins forgetting things. Sometimes they may forget several things very rapidly. When they begin to forget, you will most likely remind them, remind them again, and again, and again, etc. However, do not be surprised when they yet again forget. This is what will happen. Each day as the Alzheimer's progresses, their memories will decrease along with their ability to remember. Please do not scold the person. Chances are they will not even know, or remember, what you are scolding them for, but they will feel the emotion of your scolding them. A person with Alzheimer's may only react to your tone of voice. So, it is important to keep your voice calm and offer gentle reminders, knowing that in two minutes, you will most likely have to remind them again.

There Is No Constant Subject When Communicating With An Alzheimer's Patient

An Alzheimer's patient will say one thing and then randomly say another. It could be a statement or a question. Most often they are totally unrelated subjects. One moment they are asking for their shoes to go to a party, and they may already be wearing the shoes at the time, and in another moment they could say they want to go home to a place that once existed in their past, like say their mother's house. There is not a smooth flow of conversation, and that's okay. The important thing is to keep them as calm as possible.

Identifying Behavioral Triggers

Triggers can be identified if you pay attention to what the Alzheimer's patient is responding to. Let's go through some general triggers that can be easily identified. Triggers create an emotional response within the patient. Patients may display emotions for what appears to be no apparent reason. Let's cover the triggers according to emotional category.

Sadness – In order to identify the reason for the patient displaying sadness, listen to what they say, what they are watching, and what they are doing. If the patient is asking for a loved one and they begin to cry, we can safely assume they are sad because they miss a loved one.

Obsessive – When an Alzheimer's patient becomes obsessive; they are in actuality worrying about something. I had a patient once that would constantly ask what day it was and would begin to make a list of the days for the week. Anytime the patient found a calendar, the series of repeated questions would begin for hours. "What day is it?" Then the next question the patient would ask would be what identified the trigger. "How many days until mass?" In this case the patient was obsessing over missing mass.

Angry – When a patient displays anger, there is something that is frustrating them. One patient I had would become angry if provided a spoon, a fork and a butter knife along with dinner that required cutting, i.e. a pork chop. The patient wanted either a fork or a spoon but not both. If the patient received both, there was first frustration, then anger displayed because it would confuse the patient. This only occurred in a private setting. Later, when the patient's family made the decision to place their loved one into an Alzheimer's facility, the dining room was more open and public, as all of the patients dined together, and this particular patient was no longer getting frustrated and angry with receiving all three utensils. It's very possible that the increase in dining space helped the patient feel more relaxed and the patient most likely remembered that in restaurants, a person receives all three utensils. This patient however, had more than one trigger. And sadly, that is most often the case.

Violent – Violence in Alzheimer's patients is a subject that could use more focus. No one likes to talk about a patient with Alzheimer's becoming violent, however it happens. Patients with Alzheimer's will often have violent outbursts. One patient I had would become violent around negativity. For instance, if someone was crying and carrying on about how hopeless they felt (i.e., another patient within the facility), anger would then be displayed. The patient that had the violent outburst would attempt to harm the patient that was being negative, or in this case had depression. These outbursts occurred more than once. It was imperative to get the depressed patient away from the patient that was displaying anger. When the depressed patient was once again reassured and no longer sad, then the two patients would get along famously.

Depression – It is important to distinguish sadness from depression because they are very different. Sadness typically is displayed when a patient has a momentary sadness, which is quickly diverted with other topics. Depression is when the patient is constantly displaying sadness. Once depression is distinguished, now the need for an answer to the following question begins. "What is causing the depression?" This is where you will need to pay attention.

Example: I had a patient that was extraordinarily depressed and frequently threatened to kill herself. I would watch the other staff interact with this patient and noticed that the self-destructive behavior escalated when the staff told the patient "No, you don't want to hurt yourself." After getting some background information, I learned that this patient was walking six weeks prior and that the staff placed her in a wheelchair because she was a fall risk. She had one leg that she could not use and the other was becoming weaker. The patient kept trying to get out of the wheelchair and would repeat the phrase that would identify her trigger. "I've got to get out of here." It became clear to me that the patient felt trapped in the wheelchair. Since the patient could not walk, it became apparent to me that I needed to redirect the patients' focus. So, I began telling her to push her wheels and she could go wherever she wanted to go. Problem solved!

Fixation = An Alzheimer's Patient Distresses Over The Same Topic For A Lengthy Period Of Time

When an Alzheimer's patient fixates on something such as attending a specific function, such as church or communion, they may obsess over what day it is. Or if they don't want to be alone, or without a specific loved one, like a spouse or another relative they may have a tantrum similar to a child acting out when not getting their way. A person with Alzheimer's may also have a need to go somewhere specific like getting back home to their mothers house or even just keep moving. Some Alzheimer's patients have an aversion to sitting still, while others may sit quietly in the same place for several hours at a time.

Validating The Emotional State Of An Alzheimer's Person Is Essential

When communicating with an Alzheimer's patient, some Alzheimer's patients might say that they want to hurt themselves. This is most likely due to feeling trapped in a seemingly hopeless situation. If they are feeling trapped and say they want to kill themselves, the moment you say the words "No, you don't want to do that" is when you start the fire for the situation to escalate.

If you refuse to validate the feeling they say they have, i.e. that they indeed feel like killing themselves, by not acknowledging the feeling as real, then the person may indeed begin acting out on their statement and attempt to harm themselves.

The best thing to do in a situation like this is to validate and acknowledge the person's feelings of wanting to "get out" of the situation, keeping in mind that killing yourself is only an option when you see no other way out. So, instead of saying the words, "No, you don't want to kill yourself" which makes the patient feel as if no one is listening to how they really feel, you can ask them a question instead. One question I found incredibly helpful was asking "So when are you going to kill yourself?" The patient would then respond with "When I get around to it." which is a very good answer. The patient would then move on to a different subject and forget about killing themselves altogether because their feelings were just validated. Now the next task for you is to redirect their attention to a safe place (topic). Keep them moving!

Triggers = Words Or Actions That Draw A Negative Response From A Person With Alzheimer's. When Triggers Lead To Fixation, Validate And Question!

A person with Alzheimer's will often have a trigger. A trigger could be a spouse's name, a place they miss, or an item. When a trigger is mentioned or brought into focus, the Alzheimer's patient may begin to obsess about leaving and going to that person, place or item. They may begin crying or acting out. Once the trigger has been set in motion, it's up to you to prevent it from causing an escalation of emotional turmoil. The best way is to begin by asking random questions. This will throw off their focus. It is hard for them to tell you something when they are too busy trying to answer your questions. So constantly ask questions to redirect their thinking to a positive place or topic. They will soon forget what it was they were focusing on. Let's go over some examples.

Example One: If mass is on Sunday and the person with Alzheimer's begins to obsess with going to mass, what do you think would be the trigger? The Day! They are focused on what day it is and worrying about "missing" mass. So the trigger in this case would be a calendar and sometimes even a clock. Remove the calendar and or clock from them and you will remove the trigger. Ask them an unrelated question to throw off their focus.

11

Example Two: If an Alzheimer's patient is stressing about their situation and states that they will harm themselves. What do you think the trigger is? They feel trapped! They are looking for a way out of their situation. So their trigger is "remaining motionless". Validate their feelings by acknowledging that the feelings exist. Then help them focus on moving themselves or even pretend to move themselves' as some may be unable to do so. Encourage them! Tell them they can go wherever they want, if they are in a wheelchair, tell them to push their wheels and tell them that they are good drivers. This will entirely change their demeanor from sad and wanting to commit suicide, to a "where are we going" attitude.

If A Person With Alzheimer's Displays Violence, DO NOT Reciprocate!

A person with Alzheimer's may react to negative energy. What I mean by that phrase is this, if there is another person that is crying in the same room and is exhibiting distress, the person with Alzheimer's may display violence. The change may be instant. They may try to harm the person that is crying or displaying negative emotions. If this happens, do not yell and scream at them. Calmly walk up to them, look them in their eyes and say "It's Okay" or something similar in a calm tone of voice. This usually will calm the patient and stop them from acting out. Then quickly remove the person or thing that is generating negative energy (i.e., crying person, angry or upset person, animal or even just changing a television program, etc.)

Good Hygiene Is Often Overlooked By Alzheimer's Patients

Alzheimer's patients forget things, including how to dress and undress, shower and brush their teeth. These are simple everyday tasks that they end up no longer being able to perform. They may forget to brush their teeth or comb their hair. They may even forget to (yes I have to go there) wipe themselves after using the restroom. And they often forget to wash their hands. I have seen some patients wipe their bottom and put the tissue in their sleeve to blow their nose on later. Sad I know, but true. It is imperative to watch them closely for signs of their hygiene being neglected and get them the proper care they need. If you cannot assist them, there are several caregivers that are trained and would be willing to do so for you, either at home or in a secure facility.

Unfortunately Pets Are Often Overlooked When Their Owners Have Alzheimer's

As an Alzheimer's patient progresses through different stages of the disease, it is very common for them to overlook the basic care of not only themselves but also their pets. Food and water may be forgotten, or they may feed the pets too much. And, pets are often flea infested because nobody notices the pets when their time is devoted to the person with Alzheimer's. In many cases, a caregiver takes on this task. However, that is because a flea infestation puts the caregiver and the caregivers' home and family in a position where they too could have a flea infestation. All due to the neglect of an animal whether it's on purpose or not. It is very important to monitor the pets and their welfare, as they are innocent in these situations. Alzheimer's patients progressively forget things that seem ordinary in an everyday normal adult human life. In essence, their brain is dying little by little. And, currently, there is no cure.

A Person With Alzheimer's Often Forgets To Take, Or Takes More Medication Than They Are Supposed To

Because forgetting is part of the disease, Alzheimer's patients will oftentimes miss or overdose on their medications. This is a very important part of their life. The medications that they are given are meant to help keep them calm and in some cases have been known to slow the process of decline in brain matter. And in some cases, the medication prevents seizures. If you suspect that someone you know has been missing medications, please get them the help they need. There are several health provider options available. You may find out more about Alzheimer's at www.alz.org.

A Person With Alzheimer's Is Vulnerable And Should Have A Support System In Place To Protect Them

The very sad truth is that there are people that will try to take advantage of a person with Alzheimer's. They will get the person to give them money or steal their medications. They may even use their entire paychecks on themselves, and may even assault or further traumatize a person that has Alzheimer's. If you suspect abuse of a person with Alzheimer's, report it! Be their voice. They often do not remember, and are not even aware of, their surroundings or the people that are in their life. I practically lived with a patient for months and that patient never knew or remembered my name. It is a part of the process when their brain is deteriorating. The person may still be funny and remember many things, however they will forget or fail to remember many other things when they have Alzheimer's.

Embrace The Funny Moments! Laughter Does The Heart Good, Like A Medicine!

A person with Alzheimer's oftentimes will say or do some very funny, outrageous things. Take a moment to laugh at the situation when it warrants it. I'm not talking about laughing at a person, but with them. I will give you an example.

I was with two Alzheimer's patients one day. I will call them June and Marie. June walked up to Marie and I. The conversation went as follows.

June said to Marie "As soon as you get your shoes on we'll go to the concert."

Marie already had her shoes on and looked down at them, then back at the June, and then at me rather incredulously.

Marie then responded to the June saying, "I already have my shoes on."

June then asked the Marie "Well do you want to give them up?"

Marie responded rather emphatically to June "No. I'm not going to give you my shoes!"

By this time I am laughing hysterically and Marie is laughing right along side me, then June laughs too and steps away for a moment.
Marie's shoes were like half the size of June's.

A few moments later June again walks up to Marie and I. June says to Marie "We are going to go to the jungle."

This resulted in more laughter and additional conversation.

Believe me it can be a jungle out there. Be prepared for it!

Being A Caregiver Is A Full-Time Job

If you are a caregiver, you know very well the hectic schedule and long hours that tend to go along with the job. I know from a personal and a professional standpoint, things that you can do to help you stay alert and focused.

First is, take a deep breath! Close your eyes and think of a funny moment in your life. The one memory, that perhaps had you laughing hysterically. There! You can feel that joy again just by visiting that memory. Memories are powerful. We all should take time for ourselves to collect our thoughts and drown out all of the chaos that so regularly seems to enter our lives.

TIPS FOR CAREGIVER PROFESSIONALS

Be Firm With Your Employer Regarding The Number Of Hours You Can Work

As a professional caregiver, you know that employers will work you to the very last hour of every day, if you let them. Caregiver's are in demand, yes. However, I have noticed that employers will give one caregiver ninety hours a week, every week, and another caregiver will be scheduled for perhaps only eleven hours a week. Remember, there is always someone else to take your place! Don't fall into the trap that you are the only one that can help. There are others that are willing to fill in. If you allow an employer to continually pile hours on you, then you are walking a dangerous line. You are a valuable person, no matter how many hours you work or how many people you help. We are all human and we all require time to rest. So, put your compassion on the back burner when it comes to your schedule. When your boss schedules you for sixty to eighty hours in a single week, politely and firmly inform them that you are willing to work a set number of hours per week. Remember a full-time job stops at forty hours per week! Anything over that is overtime and you will be sacrificing yourself, and time with your family and friends, if you begin to overwork yourself. It is important that you remember that you are not saying "no" to the people who need help when you turn down hours. You are saying "yes" to not only your own well being, but to maintaining quality service which you provide when you look after a patients' well being.

Don't Take Things Personally

Oftentimes as a caregiver it is easy to fall into the schedule mode. It's all about the schedule. Well, in some cases that's very true. However, it is important that you be spontaneous at least once per week and take time for yourself, your family and/or your friends or animals. If you spend all the time you've set aside from your work schedule with family or friends, or doing household chores, it doesn't count as quality "me" time. Everyone should take a little "me" time in order to refocus and refresh. So, go to the beach, go to the shopping mall, meditate, go play golf, something! You need to interact with other people outside of your care giving duties. However, you also need to have some quality time alone.

Create A Visual Chart For Your Time!

Creating a visual chart will help you see just how much time you are giving to work, others and yourself. There are 168 hours in one week. Create a pie chart to help you get started organizing your time. A simple circle will show what your schedule is like if you spent equal time for each (56 hours for each category), compared to if you spent 81 hours working per week.

So the equal number of hours per week would be 56 hours. Remember that you require 8 hours of sleep per night, which totals 56 hours. That's 56 hours of sleep required in a week so you are subtracting the 29 hours from just your required sleep time, you will still be short 27 hours of sleep per week if you work an 81-hour week. That's some serious sleep deprivation, which is known to cause all kinds of health issues. Basically it's an accident waiting to happen. You could forget to perform a very important task, i.e. medicine reminder. And if you drive in that sleep deprived state and fall asleep at the wheel, you are putting others at risk in addition to yourself. It is equivalent to driving drunk. Please be sure to balance your rest with your work and play time to ensure the safety of not only yourself, but also the other people (including children) around you.

Do Not Argue With A Patient!

If you find yourself arguing with a patient, it is time for you to step away. Arguing with a patient is a sure sign of caregiver burnout. If it isn't dealt with appropriately in the early stages, the situation could escalate to dangerous proportions. Do everyone a favor and take some time off! No excuses! Do not yell and scream at the patient. Calmly walk up to them, look them in their eyes and say "It's okay" or something similar in a calm tone of voice. Ask and validate what it is the person wants, and try to find out the reason for their being upset. This usually will calm and stop the patient from acting out or attempting to engage in an argument.

Dress In Bright Clothing

Patients absolutely love to look at pretty things. Oftentimes caregivers fail to even put on makeup because they are so busy taking care of others, they forget about themselves. Not only will you cheer up the patient, but you will also feel yourself become more confident as your relationship with them grows. Just try it for a week and you will see the difference this one small step can make.

Have A Support System In Place

There are some people that will try to take advantage of a caregiver's good intentions. They will attempt to have caregivers' do work for free because they know there is the deep feeling of wanting to help someone else burning in your heart. Whether they are patients, clients, employers, family members or friends, know when to say "NO". Find people you can trust to help encourage you when you need it, someone who will look at the situation objectively and give you honest feedback. If you don't have someone to talk to then feel free to contact me through my website at http://elainekleid.wix.com/elaine-kleid and I will do my best to help you.

Organize Daily Tasks To Enhance Productivity

For example, you can do laundry and dishes at the same time; you can also cook simultaneously while carrying out these tasks. Start the dinner, put it in the oven or on the stove, start the washer, start the dishwasher and while all these things are going, you still have time to vacuum, dust, fluff pillows, update your log book, get the patient/client something to drink, reminding them of medications when doing so. Sounds busy, but it will take much less of a toll on you if you multi-task instead of only doing one thing at a time. You can do it!

TIPS FOR CAREGIVERS THAT ARE HELPING FAMILY AND/OR FRIENDS

Know Your Limits!

If you are caring for your parent, and there are no family members to help you, do not try to do it all alone. There are people available to help. Several caregivers are willing to work with you to reduce the cost of having a professional from a company provide for your loved one. If you find yourself overworked and reaching the boiling point, contact local services for help. They are there to help you! There are non-profit organizations that will hook you up with the right people to get you and your loved one the help you need. There is a saying "A closed mouth don't get fed". It's very true. If you don't speak up, then no one will know that you need help. It is okay to admit that you need help because everyone does. Check with the state, Alzheimers.org or the Red Cross to name a few. You could even contact some local churches that may know of someone else who could help you.

Try To Focus On Making The Situation Better And Not On How Bad It Is By Keeping Organized

The more you focus on bettering the situation and trying to refrain from being too emotional, the more positive your outlook will remain. Look to combine things that don't need to be separate. If a table would be more useful next to the patient with a port-a-potty on the opposite side, see what you can do to keep those items close to the wall, away from walkways. If someone is asking for water and you notice it is at the same time every single night, then start putting the water next to him or her when you are going in that direction with his or her dinner. Plan ahead by streamlining the tasks that you are performing. Combine them. Do several things at one time without all the labor by mapping it out. As I covered under the professional section, you can cook dinner, place it in the oven, start a load of laundry in the washer, start the dishwasher, vacuum, dust, take out the trash, etc. all while these other tasks are taking care of themselves. Organization will help you manage much more than the average person who tries to tackle only one task at a time. It will also help you focus on making the best of the situation.

Recruit Family And/Or Friends To Help You

The ideal situation would be for there to be rotating schedule if you are caring for someone at home, similar to the assisted living facilities. This of course cannot always happen, so if you've tried your best to organize and keep a smoothly running household and it is still too much, then you may want to consider an assisted living facility. If you cannot afford one, the state may intervene. Be sure someone is designated with the Power Of Attorney to make the important decisions for your loved ones if they are no longer capable of doing so on their own.

Communicate Your Emotions Effectively

If you have reached a point that you can no longer do things because you're frustrated, or you just need to talk, call someone or chat online. There are several folks available online and you are not the only one experiencing this situation! I myself experienced it as a child, and then later as an adult and professional. Please, I am asking you to make sure that you take care of you. If you don't take care of you, then you will not be able to take care of someone else. Be proactive in researching information and gathering data about the different stress relief methods. I sometimes will listen to Chakra Music. It is a simple single bowl that sets off a sound for a lengthy period of time. It helps focus on "one thing". I think sometimes with all of the distractions in this world, and particularly when dealing with a person that has Alzheimer's, that it is important to focus on one thing, just to exercise that ability to keep it working. Then when times get rough, you find it automatic to focus on making the situation better and it becomes easier to handle the trials that are sent your way.

Redirecting An Alzheimer's Patients' Focus To Prevent Violent Behavior

Once a trigger has been identified, then the diffusing of anger can occur. You must pay attention to the patients' emotional behavior, and monitor what they are doing before, during and after the demonstration of emotion, in order to properly identify the trigger(s). For sadness because they miss a loved one that passed on, rather than tell the patient "the person they miss is dead" (which could emotionally be traumatic for the patient), this is where you should redirect it to a positive. For instance, instead of commenting or reminding the patient that their loved one is deceased, focus instead on a positive experience they may have had with that particular loved one. Ask random questions that will give you insight i.e., "Did you go to school together?" could be a good start. Get the patient talking about good memories. Tell them you know that they miss their loved one and perhaps even you miss them too. But DO NOT SAY any of the following "No." or "You don't miss them." or "They are dead." It's important to keep it positive while simultaneously validating their feelings.

An example for instance is when a patient I mentioned earlier was displaying depression and stated a desire to commit suicide, the reason the violent behavior escalated when the staff would tell the patient "No" is because that patient was not feeling validated. The patient wanted recognition for the very real feelings that were being experienced. The patient felt trapped in the wheelchair and felt like they were going nowhere. So rather than saying "No" when the patient threatened suicide, I took an unorthodox approach and asked "So when are you going to kill yourself?" The patient then calmly replied, "When I get around to it." The self-destructive behavior then dissipated because the patient received validation of their feelings. Remember, with Alzheimer's patients, it's all about feelings and keeping their emotional state positive, even if you need to be a little unorthodox.

Begin Making Arrangements For Care

Provided it is within your budget, there are several companies that offer "At Home Care". However, many people cannot afford them. If that is the case in your situation, then you have the option of staying at home with your loved one and/or having someone else in your friend or family circle to help you. As the Alzheimer's progresses, it will be imperative that someone be in attendance to your loved one 24/7. The reason for this is, regular tasks will be forgotten. Tasks like going to the toilet. They may even begin to ask what a toilet is at some point. Be ready to assist them because they will need you. Oftentimes, this is where a "Power Of Attorney" contract should be drawn up designating someone to make all of the decisions regarding care and estate holdings. A person with Alzheimer's is vulnerable and should have a support system in place to protect them.

Communicating With Someone That Has Alzheimer's

As I mentioned earlier in this book, conversation with a person that has Alzheimer's would best be described as random. There usually is no set topic or flow of conversation. The person may say they miss a person one moment and begin to cry, and the next moment they may think that you are the person that they miss. And, unfortunately, it could well be you that they say they miss, even as you have stood next to that person for the entire day. If it is your mom or dad that is forgetting you, it could be painful to realize that they are forgetting who you are, or that you are even there. I myself had assisted someone that had Alzheimer's and I practically lived with him for several months. He never knew my name. He would just call me Sugar. That's also what he called his dog, Sugar. I also watched my mother forget things during my time with her. So I can relate personally and professionally to this subject.

Please know that you are not alone and there are many others who share in your pain, and can offer you strength by holding out their hand and providing you with helpful tips to ease your struggles in this often, very trying situation. But know this, all normal conversation with a person that has Alzheimer's will disappear. You will only have the moments that you share with them. Do your best to make them happy moments. Remind them of things they once thought fun. If they do remember it will make them smile. That is what is important. The smiles. Not the flow of perfect subjects or sentences, but the smiles.

Focus On Making Happy Memories!

Even though someone has Alzheimer's they don't all lose their sense of humor. Believe me, sometimes they may say something so very serious, but if you take a step back for a moment and try to put it into context it can sometimes be hilarious. Embrace these moments. I am not talking about making fun of, or laughing at the person. I am referring to laughing at the absurdities of the moment, because there will be several. The person will often laugh along with you. That is sharing a moment together. That is what you want to hold on to. Sharing very happy and funny moments that you can take with you when it comes time to let them go. Make happy moments. Do not let the repetitive reminders overwhelm you. I had a person I was providing care to repeat the word hamburger exuberantly for almost an entire day! Believe me when I say there will be repetitive moments and reminders. However, don't focus on them. Focus on the person and their mood. Try to keep it positive for them. If something upsets them, remove it. There will come a time when you may have to hide certain objects from them. Many people with Alzheimer's are notorious for putting large objects in the toilets and clogging up the plumbing. Tip: Do not keep a garbage can in your bathroom. I am speaking from experience.

Preparing For The Time You Will Need To Let Go

This is the moment you decide when the person with Alzheimer's should be placed in a nursing home or receive hospice care at home. When the person becomes unable to use the bathroom, or walk, or eat, someone will need to help them with those tasks. Hospice will keep a person as comfortable as possible until they pass away. The person with Alzheimer's must be diagnosed by their doctor as only having approximately six months or less to live for hospice to step in.

Many times the family decides to place the person with Alzheimer's in a nursing home. When this happens, the person will have others around them to socialize with. They may have friendly interactions and they may not. Do not expect the nursing home to inform you if a fistfight breaks out amongst the patients. Believe me, I know from experience. They will only neutralize the situation and that usually means more medication to keep them quiet. A nursing home still may be a better choice however given the 24 hour care and fulltime staff availability. When an Alzheimer's patient begins to display anger, it is important that everyone be safe. And, if you are the only person caring for a person with Alzheimer's, it is important that you have some backup if, or when, things get out of hand.

Because people with Alzheimer's develop what are called "Triggers" (things that set them off) it is much better to have multiple staff members present. A person with Alzheimer's in the final stages could display bouts of temper or emotional moments when they are presented with an object, hear a name or a word, and react, and not in a positive way. That is why you need to know what, where, when, who and why, so you can have the object, etc. removed and distract them by asking questions.

Conclusion

I hope you find these tips helpful when dealing with those who have Alzheimer's. Whether you're a professional caregiver or a loved one who cares, I wish you all the best and will keep you in my prayers.

And remember, there is help out there. You are not alone! Please visit www.alz.org for additional information.

I would love to hear from you, and would enjoy knowing that you find these tips helpful in your journey.

And if you have additional tips that could help someone, please share them.

Thank you.

Elaine Kleid

www.ingramcontent.com/pod-product-compliance
Lightning Source LLC
Chambersburg PA
CBHW041116180526
45172CB00001B/280